Intermittent Fasting For Women

*The Practical Essentials for Achieving
Lasting Weight Loss and Health Results
with Intermittent Fasting*

not limited to, —errors, omissions, or inaccuracies.

ISBN-13: 978-1726039178

ISBN-10: 172603917X

Table of Contents

Introduction

I want to thank you for purchasing this book, *"Intermittent Fasting for Women: The Practical Essentials for Achieving Lasting Weight Loss and Health Results with Intermittent Fasting."*

Does the title of this book make you curious? It sounds pretty nice to be able to lose weight, achieve your health goals, and maintain the weight loss, doesn't it? Not just that, you will be able to lose weight without following any of those harmful crash diets. Almost sounds too good to be true, right? Well, the good news is it's not, and you are in the right place to make it happen.

Did you know that your body is effectively fasting while you sleep? Not just that, you tend to fast in between your meals as well. Intermittent fasting is simply an extension of this period of fasting.

Do you want to learn more about the intermittent fasting lifestyle, but aren't sure where to begin? If yes, then this is the perfect book for you. Listen up, ladies—this book is for you! You can achieve your weight loss and health goals with intermittent fasting. In this book, you will learn about intermittent fasting, its effect on women, different methods of intermittent fasting, myths about intermittent fasting, eating protocols, tips to lose weight on a budget, and much more. Apart from all this, this book also contains recipes for tasty and delicious intermittent-fasting-friendly recipes. So, if you are ready, let's dive in and get started right away!

(By the way, when I use the term "diet" in this book, I am simply referring to the way in which you eat. Intermittent fasting is a lifestyle, not a short-term crash diet that sets you up for failure.)

Chapter One: About Intermittent Fasting

Intermittent fasting is a brief fast wherein you need to fast anywhere between 12 to 16 hours or more in a day. During the fasting period, you cannot consume any calories, unless the fasting method says otherwise. It probably sounds a little tricky to follow. However, your body tends to fast, regardless of whether you are doing it intentionally or unintentionally. For instance, if you have your dinner at 8 p.m. and then the next meal you consume is on the following day at noon, your body is effectively on a fast for 16 hours. Yes, you are fasting, and you are probably not even aware of it.

Did you know that this, in fact, is a popular method of intermittent fasting? Intermittent fasting probably seems slightly technical, but you have probably unknowingly followed the protocols of intermittent fasting. Before you learn about intermittent fasting, you must know the difference between fasting and fed states. Your body is in a "fed" state if you consume some food every couple of hours. While your body is in the fed state, it will digest, absorb, and assimilate nutrients from all the food that you consume. The primary priority of the body is to burn fat during this state.

Usually, most of us tend to stay in the fed state throughout the day, except when we sleep. All the benefits of an intermittent fast are because the body is in a fasted state. While in a "fasted state," your body will burn fats to provide energy. So, what is an intermittent fast? It merely means that you must fast for anywhere between 12 and 48 hours. The length of the fast is known as the "fasting window". The time when you can eat is the "eating window". Intermittent fasting oscillates between fasting and eating periods.

During your fasting window, you can consume liquids without any calories like water, herbal tea, or even some broth. It is better to avoid any calories when you fast, but you can include a couple of low-cal green vegetable juices to maintain the nutrient requirements of your body. There are no hard and fast rules when it comes to intermittent fasting, and it is subjective. If you fast for less than 24 hours, you will have an eating window. The eating window is the time at which you can eat before the fast starts.

All those who practice intermittent fasting limit their eating window to between six and 12 hours. The most common times for intermittent fasting are 12, 14, 16, and 18 hours. For instance, when you fast for 12 hours, the eating window will be 12 hours. You can start your eating window at 8 a.m. in the morning and end it at 8 p.m. at night. You can break your fast on the next day at 8 a.m.

A couple of benefits that intermittent fasting offers women are sustainable weight loss, increase in the lean muscle, better energy levels, better response to cell stress, reduction in inflammation as well as oxidative stress, better insulin sensitivity, and the triggering of the production of growth hormone. You will learn more about these benefits in the coming chapters.

Intermittent fasting is popularly known as IF, and it is an excellent method to become lean and lose weight. It also helps improve your energy levels, stamina, and cognitive functions. Intermittent fasting is a great way of life, and it offers plenty of health benefits. However, the effects that intermittent fasting has depend on biology. So, the effect it will have on men is different from its effect on women. Here comes the tricky part. Intermittent fasting has different benefits, but a woman's body is usually sensitive to signs of starvation, and therefore it works differently for women.

Fasting and Hormones

If you aren't careful while following the protocols of intermittent fasting, it can cause a hormonal imbalance in your body. A woman's body is relatively more sensitive to the signals of starvation than that of a man. So, whenever your body notices a decrease in your food intake, it tends to misinterpret this as starvation and in turn, increases the production of leptin and ghrelin. Leptin and ghrelin are the two hormones that trigger hunger. When there is an increase in the secretion of these chemical compounds, you will experience extreme hunger. Technically, your body doesn't need any extra food, but it is merely your hormones that tell you otherwise.

Whenever a woman's body feels that it is headed towards a famine (intentional or not), it increases the secretion of the hunger hormones. The hunger hormones, as is obvious from the name, signal your body to increase the intake of food. Also, if there isn't enough food to survive, then your body will start to shut down its reproductive system. A woman's body will not want to procreate when it feels like there isn't sufficient sustenance to nourish itself.

In fact, it is the body's natural defense against a potential pregnancy during famines. Your body will protect itself from pregnancy, regardless of whether you want to conceive or not. Your body cannot differentiate between a self-imposed fast and a famine. Therefore, the body cannot differentiate between starvation and intermittent fasting. Well, that's why the default protective mechanism kicks in. There are a few side effects of intermittent fasting that can lead to hormonal imbalances. The hormonal imbalances in the body can lead to metabolic stress, irregular menstrual cycles, amenorrhea in extreme cases, anxiety, depression, and can even cause other fertility issues.

All the hormones present within the body are interrelated. When there is a disruption in the level of one hormone, it will affect all the other hormones as well. All this is quite similar to a domino effect. Think of hormones as the messengers in the body that control all the various bodily functions from digestion to reproduction, from metabolism to the regulation of blood pressure, and so on. You don't want to disrupt the natural rhythm of all these functions, do you? All these drawbacks might make you wonder if you can practice intermittent fasting at all. Well, don't let these side effects scare you. If you practice intermittent fasting in a proper manner and opt for a relaxed approach, you don't have to worry about all this. When you don't fast for too long, then you can achieve your weight loss and health goals. In fact, a little caution goes a long way when it comes to intermittent fasting.

Most women tend to ignore any hunger pangs they experience. If you ignore them, these signals merely grow louder. Do you know what is worse than ignoring these hunger pangs? Being unable to ignore the cues and then binging! Never try to balance under-eating by overindulging. It will just create a vicious cycle that you cannot break easily. Also, such a pattern is bound to throw the hormonal balance in your body out of whack.

An animal study was conducted in 2013 on female rats, which showed that fasting for prolonged periods could lead to the disruption of their menstrual cycle and the shrinking of their ovaries as well. The male rats in the study experienced insomnia and a decrease in the production of testosterone. However, there are only limited human studies about the effect that intermittent fasting has on men and women. Most of the data available is from animal studies. There is one point that all these diets seem to agree with: fasting for extremely long periods leads to a hormonal imbalance in the female body. It doesn't mean that intermittent fasting is bad. In fact, there is a solution to all these problems.

Experimenting with intermittent fasting is merely a small part of your life, isn't it? For a woman, even this small experiment can have a significant impact. Hormones help regulate various functions in the body like ovulation. Ovulation is quite sensitive to the energy levels present in the body. Think of the HPG Axis or the hypothalamic-pituitary-gonadal axis as the ATC (air traffic controller) in the body. The hypothalamus secretes gonadotropin and it, in turn, releases the GnRH hormone. The GnRH hormone signals the pituitary gland to release LH (luteinizing hormone) and FSH (follicular stimulating hormone). These LH and FSH hormones act as gonads, i.e., they behave as testes or ovaries. In women, it kick-starts the secretion of estrogen and progesterone, which are important to start ovulation and sustain pregnancy. On the other hand, it triggers the flow of testosterone and sperm in male bodies. It is important to time any GnRH pulses in the body. If these pulses aren't properly timed, then it can completely disrupt the cycle in women. Apart from this, GnRH pulses are quite sensitive to various environmental factors and fasting can cause harmful alterations to them.

Well, it does sound a little worrisome, doesn't it? However, don't let all this scare you away. Learn to listen to your body and don't overdo the fast, that's about it. Follow these simple guidelines and you can follow the protocols of intermittent fasting with amazing results!

Who Can and Cannot Fast?

You can fast as long as you are a healthy adult and don't suffer from any illnesses that affect your metabolism. Anyone who doesn't fall under the following categories can follow intermittent fasting: you are pregnant, have any eating disorders or are recovering from an eating disorder, you experience chronic depression, are under extreme stress, or suffer from insomnia. The energy needs of a pregnant woman are more than that of an ordinary woman, and therefore, you must not fast if you want to start a family soon. If you think you are under chronic stress, or if you cannot sleep properly, you need to nurture your body and not put it under further stress. Also, if you struggle with an eating disorder or struggled with an eating disorder in the past, a diet that prescribes fasting will further the problem. The best thing that you can do is learn about nutrition and listen to your body. Your body knows what it needs, and you have to listen to it.

Chapter Two: Benefits Of Intermittent Fasting

With intermittent fasting you oscillate between periods of eating and fasting. There are several benefits this diet offers, and there are scientific studies as well as research that support these claims. In this section, you will learn about the different benefits this way of life offer.

Weight Loss

The main reason that many people take up intermittent fasting is to help them lose weight. Intermittent fasting, particularly when combined with sensible exercise, is a powerful tool in the fight against the obesity epidemic that is sweeping the world.

There are endless examples of people who have successfully lost weight (and kept it off) while on a program of intermittent fasting. Sometimes efforts to reduce weight, even if they use intermittent fasting, are unsuccessful. There are many reasons for this such as hormonal imbalance, stress, poor sleep, and even prescription drugs. Despite these problems, intermittent fasting is a beneficial strategy for losing weight. But if you find that you are unsuccessful at losing weight when intermittent fasting or otherwise, then you may be well advised to seek medical help.

https://www.ncbi.nlm.nih.gov/pubmed/12425705

https://www.ncbi.nlm.nih.gov/pubmed/15640462

Sleep

In the paragraph above, it was mentioned that sometimes efforts to lose weight are undermined by insufficient sleep.

There has been at least one scientific study which has shown that people who persist with intermittent fasting for a year or more have better sleep. The reasons why this occurs are no doubt complicated, but there's been conclusive demonstrations that intermittent fasting over an extended period assists good sleep.

Mood and Motivation

The study of the effect of intermittent fasting on mood and motivation is in its infancy. There is a lack of research on large populations, using the statistical techniques of randomized controls. However, some studies have demonstrated that intermittent fasting does improve both mood and motivation in a surprisingly short period. As there is profound controversy about the pharmacological treatments of people's mental state, any treatment which has no side effects and many potential benefits must be considered seriously.

Cardiovascular Health

Intermittent fasting leads to a reduction in weight. For this and other reasons, it leads to an improvement in cardiovascular health. The cause of such disease is usually atherosclerosis, the deposit of plaque in blood vessel walls. The dysfunction of the endothelium, which is a thin lining of the blood vessels, causes atherosclerosis. A healthy endothelium works to prevent this insidious deposit. The endothelium is not doing its job properly if plaque builds up. Obesity, especially where the fat deposits are in the abdominal area, leads in many cases to this buildup of plaque.

Other causes of this deposit are stress and inflammation. Intermittent fasting assists in the reduction of these, as well as obesity. Some studies show improvements in all risk factors for cardiovascular health.

Gut Health

Increasingly, scientists are becoming ever more aware that microorganisms living in the human gut or digestive system perform vital functions. These are known as the microbiome. There are trillions of them and they are in other parts of the body, apart from the gut. Many diseases originate in the gut, not only illnesses concerning that part of the body, but also of the brain, the heart, and all other regions of the body.

There is research on mice that caloric restriction improves that part of the microbiome in the gut. The effect of this is to prolong the life of the mice. In humans, the effects of dietary changes are very swift, even as short as hours. Studies are currently being done to verify that the real effects of intermittent fasting observed in the gut health of mice are true for humans as well.

Brain

Research has shown that the reduction in calorie intake of intermittent fasting has beneficial effects on the brain. Intermittent fasting results in something called brain-derived neurotrophic factor (BDNF) that improves the means by which the brain neurons resist degeneration and dysfunction.

A consequence of intermittent fasting on the brain is that it boosts its power. The fasting triggers a mild stress reaction in the brain, which makes it more active. Scientists explain this by the evolution of the brain in prehistoric times, which conditioned it to become more active when food was needed.

Studies with rats have shown that intermittent fasting can

prevent the onset of memory problems for times equivalent to at least 20 years in human beings. Studies throughout the world confirm that these positive results for intermittent fasting by rats apply to people who practice intermittent fasting.

https://www.ncbi.nlm.nih.gov/pmc/articles/PMC2622429/

Neurodegenerative Diseases

This term may seem a bit strange to most people, but what follows may help. Two well-known neurodegenerative diseases are Alzheimer's disease and Parkinson's disease. Alzheimer's is a fatal condition in which a person's memory is progressively destroyed by the illness. Famous individuals who have had it include the great U.S. President Ronald Reagan and the well-known singer Glenn Campbell.

Parkinson's disease is also severe; it is a disease of the nervous system whose symptoms include tremors and slow movements. It affects older people such as evangelist Billy Graham and famous singer Linda Ronstadt. Unlike Alzheimer's, Parkinson's, although debilitating, is not always fatal.

There is research to show that lowering the intake of energy by fasting often, at least twice a week, may assist the brain in avoiding neurodegenerative diseases such as Alzheimer's and Parkinson's. Some may ask, "Why not just reduce the amount of food eaten?" A smaller food intake is of less or no benefit because the glycogen stored as a result of this eating may not be used for up to 12 hours.

Eating three meals a day, with snacks in between, does not give the body the chance to deplete the resulting glycogen. Fasting is a way in which the body has to practice autophagy (self-eating of cells). It won't do this if there is glycogen present as an energy source.

http://www.aging-us.com/article/NjJf3fWGKw4e99CyC/text

https://www.ncbi.nlm.nih.gov/pubmed/17306982

Diabetes

Diabetes, by itself, is a severe condition and is often a precursor to serious cardiovascular diseases such as heart attack and stroke. The cause of diabetes is the buildup of glucose in the blood. Diabetes occurs when the body is resistant to insulin. Intermittent fasting reduces the buildup of glucose (blood sugar) and substantially lowers insulin resistance. Intermittent fasting is an excellent protection against the onset of diabetes.

Inflammation

We are all familiar with the inflammation that occurs in throat glands when you have the flu, or the inflammation around a scab as a cut heals. This inflammation is a part of the body's way of dealing with real damage.

Unfortunately, not all inflammation is good; inflammation is often the cause of many serious problems such as diabetes, atherosclerosis, and neurodegenerative diseases. This sort of inflammation is called chronic inflammation. It occurs when the body is unable to remove the source of irritation. Research has shown that the modern lifestyle, with its excess sugar, processed food, chronic stress, and lack of exercise is often to blame for chronic inflammation.

Researchers at Yale University have discovered that a compound produced by the body during intermittent fasting wards off the inflammatory response in many situations where it is not needed and can cause damage.

https://www.hindawi.com/journals/bmri/2014/761264/

Autoimmune Diseases

These are quite common, even though they are not as well-known as they probably must be. They affect about 50 million people in the USA alone and many hundreds of millions of others in the rest of the world. The cause is the body's immune system, which works to protect it against foreign intruders, turning on healthy cells in different ways. There are more than 80 autoimmune diseases; some of the most common are rheumatoid arthritis, celiac disease, (gluten intolerance) and psoriasis, a skin condition which affects many. Intermittent fasting has been shown to be beneficial to the sufferers of many autoimmune diseases.

https://www.ncbi.nlm.nih.gov/pubmed/11220789

Pain

As mentioned above, intermittent fasting has been proven to assist in significantly reducing inflammation. One of the benefits of this reduction in inflammation is a decrease in pain. There have been many reports of different sorts of pain reduction as a consequence of intermittent fasting.

Skin

One of the benefits of intermittent fasting is usually an improvement in the quality of the skin. The reason for this is that, when fasting, the body's cells have a reduction in the aging process. We shall have more to say about the effect of intermittent fasting on aging near the end of this chapter.

What about diseases of the skin? Research has shown that

intermittent fasting had a very positive effect on 80 percent of psoriasis sufferers. Other dangerous conditions of the skin which benefit from intermittent fasting are contact dermatitis, acne, and eczema.

Cancer

The very word "cancer" terrifies most people. There are many sorts of this disease, some far more virulent than others, and it is unlikely that there will ever be one single cure for all cancers. Although it is not a cure, intermittent fasting helps to prevent cancer. It contributes to reducing the very adverse effects of modern treatments such as chemotherapy.

https://www.ncbi.nlm.nih.gov/pubmed/16126250

All these benefits help increase your lifespan and help you lead a healthier life. Not only will you lose weight, but you can also improve your overall health if you follow intermittent fasting.

Chapter Three: Methods Of Fasting

There are different variations of intermittent fasting, and in this section you will learn about the best methods of intermittent fasting for women.

Crescendo Fasting

Intermittent fasting is a simple fasting protocol, but it can be slightly hard on your body if you are new to it or if you jump in way too quickly. So, listen up, ladies, if you are new to intermittent fasting, then the best method of fasting is crescendo fasting. In this method of fasting, you fast for a couple of days a week instead of daily. It is the best form of intermittent fasting and is a gentle approach that will enable your body to get used to fasting gradually. A radical approach will not do your body any good, and you need to start slowly. You can obtain all the benefits of intermittent fasting without causing any harmful hormonal imbalances in your body. When you follow the protocols of this diet properly, you can shed all the excess pounds you want to. You can follow any of the other approaches as well if you aren't new to fasting.

The rules of this fast are quite simple. You can fast for two or three days in a week and make sure that you don't fast on any another days. For instance, you can fast on Tuesday, Thursday, and Saturday. On the days you fast, keep your exercise protocol light and do some basic cardio or even some yoga. Make sure that your fasting period doesn't exceed 12-16 hours. The days when you don't fast, and you want to take up any high-intensity exercises, you must eat normally to maintain your energy levels. Always keep your body hydrated, and you can even have calorie-free beverages on your fasting days. If you decide to fast for two days a week, after two weeks, you can add another day. However, you must not exceed three days a week and the fasting days must never be consecutive. If you want to, you can have about five to eight grams of branched-chain amino acids (BCAAs) on the days you fast. These will help provide additional energy on the days you fast and reduce hunger pangs and fatigue.

16/8 Method

This is also popularly known as the Lean gains method. It is a short routine of intermittent fasting that will help you to burn body fat and improve your lean muscle. In this diet, you have to fast for 16 hours daily, and your eating window is restricted to eight hours a day. For instance, you can start your fast at 7 p.m. and then fast until 11 a.m. the following day. So, you can break your fast with a meal at noon and end with a meal at night before 7 p.m. If you start your fast on Monday night, it will extend until noon on Tuesday and so on. You can move on to this method of fasting after your body gets used to the previous method of fasting.

This variant of intermittent fasting is quite simple. It can be as simple as skipping your breakfast instead of having your first meal at noon. Most of us tend to lead busy lives, and hardly any of us have the time to eat breakfast. Yes, it is as simple as that. Skip your breakfast, have a nutritious lunch, a snack, and end your day with a nutritious dinner. You cannot have any snacks post-dinner, and no more late-night snacks. It will also help regulate the circadian rhythm of your body. If you have dinner at 7:00 or 8:00 at night, you give your body sufficient time to digest the food before you go to bed.

24-Hour Protocol

It is also known as the Eat-Stop-Eat diet. As the name suggests, in this variation of intermittent fasting, you need to fast for 24 hours at a stretch. However, you must not fast more than twice a week. You can start with one day and, after a while, increase to two days a week. As mentioned, you must never fast on two consecutive days. You can select your fasting window, and you need to stick to it. You can start your fast at 8 p.m. and end it at 8 p.m. on the following day. For instance, if you start your fast at 8 p.m. on Monday night, then you can break your fast at 8 p.m. Tuesday. You can fast on Monday and Wednesday. You need to fast for 24 hours a day. Therefore, you will not have an eating window during this fast. While you fast, you can have plenty of calorie-free beverages. So, you can have your coffee, but don't add any sugar, cream, or milk to it. Herbal teas and water must be your go-to drinks. If you want, you can even spruce up your regular drinking water by adding a couple of slices of lemon and sprigs of mint to it.

5:2 Diet

The 5:2 diet is also known as the Fast Diet, and in this diet, you need to fast for two days a week. You might wonder what the difference is between this diet and the crescendo method. Unlike the crescendo method, on the days you fast, you cannot exceed 500 calories. In the crescendo method, you are free to eat after your fasting window ends. However, in this method, you can eat throughout the day, but you have a caloric restriction to follow. So, you will have to consume 500 calories twice a week and eat properly on rest of the days. You fast for two days and eat like usual on the other days of the week. You must never fast on consecutive days. If you want, you can have one 500-calories meal while you fast, or break it up into smaller meals. It is a safe method to diet and you can even start with this method if you want to.

There are a couple of general rules that you need to keep in mind when you decide to follow any of the intermittent fasting protocols. You must never fast for more than 24 hours at any given point in time. An ideal fast can last between 12 to 16 hours and nothing beyond it. Never fast on consecutive days. During the initial days of fasting, you must never fast for more than two or three days, even if the fasting window doesn't exceed 16 hours on a fasting day. Keep your exercise schedule quite light on the days of fast and keep your body thoroughly hydrated.

Chapter Four: Tips to Stay Motivated

The main reason why most diets fail is lack of motivation and creating a habit. Most people tend to start a diet with a lot of motivation, and then, as time passes by, this motivation starts to fade away. Motivation also starts to fade away when you don't get the results you expected or you don't get them soon. The results you hoped from a diet will take a while, and this causes your motivation level to take a nosedive. The one thing that you must remember is that you won't get any instant results. No diet provides you with instantaneous results and it is not good for you in the long run. Did you gain those extra 10 pounds overnight? No, you didn't. So what makes you think that you will be able to shed them overnight? It takes a while. This doesn't mean that the diet isn't working. It simply means that it will take a while to tone your body. You will not be able to achieve the perfect body that you hoped for in a week's time. A diet, when combined with exercise, provides you with the results you hoped for, after a while. It takes time. So be patient with your body, and don't give up.

At times, it really does get difficult to keep going. There may be some temptation lurking around the corner or you may simply feel disheartened. Regardless of what the reason is, here are three things that you can do to make sure that you stay motivated.

You can start off by making use of the mirror, and not the scale, to judge your progress. As you start your diet, stand in front of the mirror right after taking a shower. A full-length mirror is ideal. Notice the areas where you want to lose weight and the places where you want well-sculpted muscles.

Capture a mental picture of yourself. This will be your "before the diet" body and you can watch it change as you start following the diet. Why don't you take a picture of yourself and keep this in view to motivate yourself every time you feel like giving up? It will serve as a reminder to stay on track. It will also work as positive encouragement for you. You can gauge your progress by comparing yourself to the image. This will definitely make you want to keep going. You may not lose weight immediately, but you will be able to slowly see the fat giving way to lean muscle.

It will be helpful if you can start the diet with a partner. It can be your friend, your spouse, or even a family member. You can do the diet with them, using each other as a coach and a support system. You can fast together and exercise together. Whenever you feel like giving up, there will be someone else to keep you motivated and make sure that you are on the right track. It is simpler to shop for groceries and plan your meals when you have company.

Make sure that you include a variety of foods in your diet. No one likes to eat the same thing every single day. It gets boring and repetitive. Keep researching to find healthier alternatives. There are millions of healthy recipes available online and you can make use of them. You can also share and trade recipes. Modify them to suit your needs and requirements. If the food starts to become boring, you will lose the motivation to continue.

As a bonus tip, always keep in the forefront of your mind the reason these changes are important to you. Some call it your "why". Write it down on paper and keep it out where you can see it constantly. This will be a continual reminder to you if you're faced with a decision that may throw you off track.

Lastly, be kind to yourself if you do slip up. Don't let it derail
you completely.

Chapter Five: Things To Expect

In this section, you will learn about the different things that you can expect when you start the diet.

It's Mostly in The Mind

Intermittent fasting is very simple because, really, you don't need to count calories or prepare many meals. In fact, you don't even have to eat upon waking up if you don't want to. At least that's how many people do it. But that's not to say it's easy; it is generally very hard. And most of the challenge comes from the mind. Part of the mental challenge is thinking:

How will I be able to function well the whole day at work or school if I don't eat enough or at all?

What if I feel lightheaded due to starvation and faint?

What if I get sick as a result?

Most people who have successfully incorporated intermittent fasting in their lives had similar thoughts at first, which they were able to eventually overcome when they realized that nothing happened even if they worried about it—life went on as usual.

Mindsets are very powerful barriers, particularly ones that stick to the belief that you need to eat frequently, that breakfast is the stuff that champions are made of, and that going hungry is evil. All of that is in the head—your head. Chances are, you just believe it and haven't really experienced the truth of those statements. You may be simply mentally programmed.

One Day at a Time

If you start off with the intention of doing intermittent fasting for the rest of your life, it will seem like a little too much. Instead, do this one day at a time. It won't take you—and your body—long to find out that only being able to eat during a set window of time isn't so bad. Once you have done the first day, the next one will seem easier. And the one after that will be easier still. Before you know it, you will be full swing into an intermittent fasting regime without even noticing any difference.

Think Long-Term

Oftentimes, we tend to look at the things we do on a short-term basis, i.e., hourly or daily. For successful intermittent fasting, its best to plan on a weekly basis instead of daily or, God forbid, hourly. An example is protein. When fasting intermittently, you don't have to worry about downing a protein shake within the golden three-hour window after working out, but within 24 hours, which makes it more practical and convenient.

One of the best things about intermittent fasting is that it totally debunks the myth perpetuated by most food and supplement manufacturers: that you need to eat every few hours for optimal health and fitness. Simply put, do you really think your body cares whether or not you eat every three hours or just once or twice a day, within a particular feeding window, as long as it gets the calories it needs? I thought so.

Thinking longer-term—or slightly longer-term, at least—helps you realize that you don't need to micromanage your time and that the difference between eating all throughout your waking hours and eating within a limited period of time every day isn't that significant over the long-term. It also helps you achieve your desired ripped condition much faster.

Work Out your Goals

Before you begin, determine exactly what your goals are. If you want to change your body composition by increasing muscle mass and decreasing body fat, give the 16/8 method a go. If you are looking at anti-aging and preventing disease, do a 24-hour or a 36-hour fast once a week. No matter what you do, do not fast for more than 72 hours.

Build Your New Regime Around Your Social Life

If you do your intermittent fast between 9:30 a.m. and 5:30 p.m., the normal working day, it will not really work. For a start, you might be tempted to eat more, and second, you will cheat more often. Consider your social life and make it easy on yourself—set your feeding period to something like 12 p.m. to 8 p.m. You will find it much easier to stick to and even when you go out for a meal with friends, it won't be an issue for you.

Drink Water First Thing in the Morning

If a good deal of your fasting period is overnight, while you sleep, and it doesn't end until, say, 2 p.m. the following afternoon, the best way to stop yourself from feeling hungry is to drink a big glass of water as soon as you wake up. Overnight, your body dehydrates, and replenishing that water first thing will go a long way towards knocking hunger pangs on the head.

Drink Tea and Coffee

When your fasting period encompasses a morning, drink some tea or coffee. Provided you are not adding any cream or sugar to it, you are not breaking your fast. Drink it warm and drink it black; this will help you to focus better and will get rid of those hunger pangs. Some people advocate starting the day with something like Bulletproof® coffee, which contains MCT oil and butter. It is a very high-calorie drink but the body can easily burn these calories off as energy, and the coffee will not cause any disruption to your body's normal functions, like the repair of your cells.

Keep in Mind That You Won't Always be Hungry

The hunger hormones are activated through habit, more than as a genuine feeling of hunger. After about four weeks on an intermittent fasting regime, your body will get the message that you are not hungry when you are fasting and the hunger hormone secretion will slow down. Hunger pangs will begin to slow down in the first week and, from a psychological point of view, the thought that you will not always be hungry is a great start.

Losing Weight Isn't So Hard

When you get used to eating less frequently, your body tends to generally eat less all throughout. And the natural result is, unless you strategically want to bulk up, fat or weight loss. Try as you might to eat bigger meals, you may be pleasantly surprised to find that it becomes more and more of a challenge because your body and your mind will generally become accustomed to less food all day.

As such, intermittent fasting is both a very practical and effective option for fat loss. It provides a very simple way of cutting down on total calories without even having to change your general diet. Even if you get used to eating one or two big meals every day, those may not be enough to compensate for the loss of calories from the single meal you cut out. Essentially, cutting off one meal and eating a bit more on the remaining ones is often enough to create a significant caloric deficit for fat loss.

If you're the type who can't start the day without a glass of juice or cup of coffee, don't worry. You don't need to ditch it while fasting intermittently. Just make sure you stay under 50 calories throughout the day, which is the limit for being in a fasting state. The exact principle behind this isn't clear, but with enough reputable experts saying this, it's enough for me to roll with it. If you'll be having coffee or tea, stick to pure and unsweetened ones.

Train Less, Maximize Benefits

Oftentimes, potency requires minimalism. Much like the strength of coffee or any alcoholic drink dissipates as you dilute it with water, the efficacy of your workouts during intermittent fasting may follow suit if you train too much. But how does overtraining look in this context?

The obvious examples are exercising at a very high intensity and for longer periods of time. When you exert too much effort (intensity) than what your body can currently handle under a fasting state, you run the risk of burning out, getting sick, or being injured. Even at the right intensity, regularly working out significantly longer than what your body can safely handle runs the same risk as excess intensity. Can you imagine if you do both at the same time?

What does the right intensity look like? Generally speaking, you'll feel very uncomfortable—lightheaded, very tired and weak, or have prolonged muscle soreness—during or after working out if you overtrain. A relatively objective way of determining if you're exercising at a moderate intensity, which is ideal, is through the talk test. If you can still carry on a normal conversation while working out, albeit with some difficulty— that's moderate. If you're able to carry on a conversation in the same manner as you would over coffee with a friend, or if you can barely say a word while catching your breath, then you are under (low intensity) or over (high intensity) training, respectively.

A good way to focus your training is to prioritize compound exercises, i.e., those that involve the most number of major muscle groups to execute the movements. Examples of these are burpees, which utilize most of the major muscle groups.

Another way of prioritizing your exercise is to choose those that utilize the biggest muscle groups, particularly legs and back. Why? The bigger the muscles, the more calories required to contact them. That's why doing 1,000 crunches isn't enough to get you ripped but running daily for at least 30 minutes, which involves the biggest muscle group—the legs—can help you do so.

Choose an Indulgent Day

Some people like to have a cheat day and eat whatever they want. While you need to do this sensibly, you can have days where you eat more carbohydrates and calories—just choose cleaner food sources, like sweet potatoes, almond butter, and dark chocolate.

Keep Busy During a Fasting Period

This is one of the biggest reasons why it is easier to have your fasting period run overnight, because you are sleeping and not thinking about eating. If you are awake, keep busy; occupy yourself with something. When you first start this regime, you are not going to help yourself if all you are thinking about is the fact that you can't eat for so many hours!

Chapter Six: When And What To Eat

In this section, you will learn about when and what to eat when you fast. If you know the answer to this, then you can make the most of intermittent fasting. There aren't any hard and fast rules about intermittent fasting, and one of the best features of this diet is the flexibility that it offers. You can eat the food that you like, and you will not feel that you are on a constant "diet." The phrase "food you like" doesn't refer to all sorts of unhealthy treats, however, and you must show some prudence when it comes to what you eat.

When to Eat on a Fast Day?

For a lot of people, fasting all day long and having a good meal in the evening is the best plan for a fast day. If your calorie allowance is around 500 calories on a fasting day, then you can have one meal that's worth 500 calories at the end of the day. You also have the option of having mini-meals all throughout the day, as long as you stick to the caloric restriction. If you follow the crescendo method of fasting, then you will fast on two or three days of the week and eat like you usually do on all the other days. On the days that you fast, you can eat after your fasting window ends. It means that you can eat after you complete 12-16 hours of fasting. After you break your fast, you can have a light meal and follow it later with one or two meals.

As mentioned, there are different forms of fasting that you can follow. Select one that suits your needs. If you like to have a heavy dinner, then you can save up your calories from the rest of the day and indulge yourself at night. A lot of people find it easier to wait until the evening to have a proper meal. If you fall into this category, then do so. When you fast, you can have a couple of calorie-free snacks or maybe one low-cal bite, if you want to. If you think you can do without the snack, then please do so! When you fast throughout the day, you might notice that your body is running low on fuel. In such a case, you can have a salty snack like a handful of popcorn! You can have a small bite during your fast, and it will not break your fast unless you want it to. Make sure that you drink plenty of water throughout the day. You can include a couple of cups of herbal tea or broth as well.

You need to remember that, with intermittent fasting, you can make your own rules. If you think you cannot fast all day long, you don't have to. You might like to have dinner and breakfast the following day, and you can. You don't have to worry about breaking any rules here. It is up to you and your comfort level.

What to Eat on a Fast Day?

Well, how can you make the most of your meals on a fast day? If all you can eat on a fast day is 500 calories, then make sure that you have as much protein and fiber as you can. If you follow a method of crescendo fasting, or the Leangains method, then make sure that you eat at least 1200 calories and don't go beyond 1500 calories. You can have two hearty meals within this calorie restriction. You don't have to be afraid to fill up with lean proteins like fish, eggs, and chicken. You can even have lots of salad and vegetables too. It is quite easy to fast once you get used to it.

Food list

There are some people that advocate eating proteins, fruits, and vegetables while on a fast, but, technically speaking, you are not fasting if you are eating anything. Even having a cup of tea with honey in it can be classified as breaking the fast. However, just because you can't eat anything doesn't mean that you must avoid drinking tea. The most important thing to drink during a fast is water, at least eight glasses per day as a minimum. Not only does this keep you hydrated, it can also help you to feel fuller. Other drinks that don't contain any calories at all are black tea, black coffee, green tea, herbal teas, and carbonated water.

Do try to keep your caffeine intake down as low as you can, no more than two cups per day; too much is not good for you on an empty stomach and won't make you feel any better about not eating.

Watch out for the extra calories in milk and sugar. It might seem like a tough call to drink your morning coffee black but you will get used to it, especially when you start to see the benefits of your intermittent fasting regime kicking in. Adding a bit of cream here, a spot of sugar there, or even a bit of honey can have the effect of breaking the fast and sending your insulin levels back up. That means your body is not getting the full benefit of the fast. If you are doing a 24-hour fast, keep in mind that this is only for one or two days of the week, so be strong about it and push on. You can do it if you really want to.

When you first start an intermittent fasting regime, you may suffer from headaches. This is not dehydration (unless you are not drinking sufficient water). Instead, it is a symptom of withdrawal.

There is another good reason to watch your caffeine intake—caffeine is a diuretic and, unless you are regularly topping up with water, all those extra trips to the bathroom will take their toll. You may also suffer from a caffeine headache.

Avoid anything that is going to cause your insulin levels to spike. You know by now that insulin regulates how much fat is stored in your body, so keeping it low while you do your fast ensures that your body is able to release the fat stores, so they can be used, instead of continuing to add to them. The places where this fat is deposited are in your stomach, bottom, thighs, arms, and hips.

Some people advocate eating sugar-free gum while on a fast and the idea behind that isn't all that stupid. After all, as a human race, we have been chewing leaves and gum tree sap for many thousands of years. However, on a fast, you need to avoid all forms of chewing gum.

The regular type contains both sugar and calories, being sweetened, usually, with corn syrup. Corn syrup is a sugar form that you know better as glucose. Every time you eat a piece of this gum, your blood sugar levels rise. The sugar-free kind isn't much better because of the artificial sweeteners in it. A certain percentage of the population has an intolerance to something called phenylalanine, which is found in aspartame and can cause a lot of health problems. Avoid it altogether.

The same goes for diet drinks, whether it's a can of diet soda or a cup of diet iced tea. Steer clear of these altogether while you are fasting. While a can of diet soda, or a stick of sugar-free gum, for that matter, don't have many calories, once again it comes down to the harmful chemicals that are in them and the negative effect they will have on your health.

Diet soda has also been shown to actually raise insulin levels, which is the opposite of what you want.

Although one of the biggest benefits of fasting is the weight loss, it is also a good time to give your body a rest from the chemicals that are in so many of the foods that we eat on a daily basis. When it comes time to do a fast day, give the fake a rest and treat your body to a diet of fresh, clean water, black coffee, and unsweetened teas.

At the end of the day, it is pretty simple to work out what you can and can't consume on a fasting day. If you have to ask yourself whether you can or can't have it, the answer is to steer clear of it. It's only for a set period of time, and it will do you no end of good to give your body that break.

Chapter Seven: Myths About Intermittent Fasting

There are a lot of misconceptions that are associated with this diet, and in this section, we will bust these myths.

Myth #1: Lose weight without a calorie deficit

Explanation: When you don't eat for long periods of time, your body starts to burn fat as fuel. When you fast, it increases the levels of insulin sensitivity. That, in turn, helps store less fat. So it will seem as if you can lose fat by fasting for a few hours and build muscle while you are eating. This idea is slightly problematic because your total caloric intake for the day gradually evens out. If you eat enough during your feed times, you will replace the body fat lost during the fasting state. If you want to lose weight, then your body needs to be on a caloric deficit.

Myth#2: Lose fat and bulk up simultaneously

Explanation: There is almost no scientific evidence that supports this theory. Of course, intermittent fasting does help you lose weight, but that is only during the period where you are in a fasting state. Moreover, if you adopt the alternate day intermittent fasting method, you will lose less muscle mass than if you adopt the daily method. A complete beginner or novice will do well to first try the alternate method. That will help you lose body fat and build muscle, but not at the same time.

Myth#3: Alternative to snacking all day long

Explanation: Some people believe that they need to eat six or seven small meals a day. Or eat three large ones and two small ones and so on. Self-styled dieticians go around advocating these ideas to people who are desperate to lose weight. Nowadays, the trend is reversing, with diet books proclaiming that a large number of small meals per day is not good for health. If you find that such an arrangement suits your health requirements, by all means, go for it. Snacking on unhealthy food items during the day is the result of constant hunger brought on by unwise diets. Intermittent fasting is not a diet. It is simply the rearrangement of your eating schedules. You get to eat good, wholesome food whenever you sit down for a meal; only the meal frequency changes. Therefore, intermittent fasting is by no means an alternative to snacking.

Myth#4: It is not meant for women

Explanation: There is some scientific evidence behind the theory that women don't respond as well to fasting as men do. One study found that alternate intermittent fasting decreased the glucose tolerance levels in women and their sugar processing abilities. It increased their hunger levels and made it difficult for them to stick to the diet schedule. But there is no evidence that intermittent fasting is dangerous for women. Some more studies have shown that, while certain women display negative reactions to a fasting state, it works just fine with other women. It is simply a question of individual desires and willpower.

Chapter Eight: Tips and Tricks

When to Eat and Not What to Eat

This diet doesn't place any caloric constraint on those who follow it. The plans for this diet can be personalized quite easily. It focuses more on the time at which you can eat and not what you eat. The food doesn't matter. What matters is that you adhere to the fasting window.

This diet might not work for everyone. Don't get disheartened; you can try a different variation of the same diet. Also, before you get started with this diet, you must consult your physician or your doctor.

Stop Freaking Out!

You will have to get rid of your thoughts about the number of hours you can fast. Stop asking yourself if you can only fast for nine hours instead of ten hours! Stop worrying about how consuming a single French fry during your fasting period is going to affect it. Please relax! You have an extremely smart body, which will adapt itself to any changes you may make to your lifestyle.

If you are looking at consuming lunch or breakfast one day and want to skip it the next, go ahead! If you are aiming to become an athlete or aiming towards becoming strong and muscular, you will need to be very rigid with respect to your diet. Otherwise, you can just relax!

Do Not Worry About People Staring

You may have just begun the fast and probably notice others staring weirdly at you. You will probably go out for lunch with a couple of friends and hey, you have stopped eating lunch. Now what do you tell your friends? They will definitely ask you tons of questions; they are your friends, after all! You will probably have to take a lot of time to explain yourself, but if they do not understand what you are saying, then embrace the weirdness!

Keep Yourself Busy

If you have just started your intermittent diet, you will probably have trouble trying to curb your thoughts about hunger. You may sit around and begin to wonder about how hungry you are and will probably crave for some form of food. So let me give you a certain pattern that you can use during the first few days of your fast!

Right before the first few hours of your fast, you must consume a huge meal! An extremely huge meal. Let us call it a monster meal. You will stop worrying about when you are going to eat next! You can try to sleep for a decent amount of time, since you don't have to worry about hunger when you are dreaming! Try to keep yourself busy during the day, to avoid worrying about your hunger. Last, but never least, keep telling yourself that you do not need to think about hunger since you are a strong person!

You Can Consume Beverages, With No Calories

Yes, you have been asked to fast. But, this does not mean that you cannot drink water! All you have been told is to avoid consuming any food with calories in it! You can drink green tea in the morning and even during your fasting period if you want to. You can drink black tea or coffee during your fasting period. Always keep it simple!

Always Listen to Your Body

Each person has a different response to intermittent fasting.

You will never be able to gauge how your body will react to the fasting by comparing yourself with people around you. You need to see how your body is reacting and make the changes required.

Are you concerned about having lost too much muscle mass? For this, you will need to start keeping a track of your strength by undertaking strength training routines to assess the intensity of your strength. You can buy fat calipers that will help you track how well the fat has started to burn in your body! Always keep a track of your caloric intake! You will be able to see how your body has started to change with respect to the quantity of food you eat.

Do Not Expect to See Miracles!

This is a mistake that every beginner makes when he or she starts any fast. You will want to see results in a week or two. But what they forget is that a fast is not the only thing that will help. You need to understand the fact that there are many other factors that will affect the way you lose weight, or even the amount of weight you will lose. You have to look at intermittent fasting, along with other healthy habits, like exercise and sleep, which will ensure that you lose weight consistently.

Motivate Yourself

Above, you have been told that you must not expect miracles. Well, this may seem easy, but you will start feeling terrible when you find no changes after a week or two. This is when you will need to motivate yourself and tell yourself that you are doing a great job. You have to keep forging ahead and need to give yourself the strength to stick to the diet. You can always have a buddy with you who will help you, but if such a person does not exist, you will need to push yourself forward!

Chapter Nine: Recipes for Weight Loss

Berry Yogurt

Serves: 4

Ingredients:

- 12 ounces frozen mixed berries of your choice, thawed
- 1 ounce flaked almonds, toasted
- 24 ounces fat-free yogurt

Method:

1. Using four glasses, or Mason jars, make alternating layers of berries and yogurt.
2. Garnish with almond flakes and serve.

Detox and Fast Smoothie

Serves: 1

Ingredients:

- 1 ripe tomato

- ☐ 1/2 cup English cucumber cubes

- ☐ 1/2 stalk celery

- ☐ A bit of hot red pepper (optional)

- ☐ 2-3 cups beets

- ☐ 1/4 cup fresh cilantro

- ☐ 1/4 cup fresh parsley

- ☐ 1/2 sweet red bell pepper

- ☐ 1 small carrot, chopped

- ☐ 3 tablespoons frozen peas

- ☐ 4-5 leaves fresh spinach

- ☐ 1 tablespoon lemon juice

- ☐ A pinch salt

- ☐ 3-4 tablespoons water or coconut water

Method:

1. Add cucumber into a blender and blend until smooth.

2. Add tomato, cilantro, spinach, parsley, carrot, beet, celery, hot pepper, if using, and salt, and blend until smooth.

3. Add frozen peas, coconut water, and pepper and blend until smooth.

4. Pour into a tall glass. Stir in the lemon juice and serve.

Chestnut Mushroom Omelet

Serves: 2

Ingredients:

- ☐ 2 large eggs

- ☐ 1.8 ounces chestnut mushrooms, cleaned, finely sliced

- ☐ 2 small bunches chervil, rinsed, finely chopped

- ☐ Cracked black pepper to taste

- ☐ 4 dessert spoons organic plain yogurt

- ☐ 3 teaspoons olive oil

- ☐ 2 small cloves garlic, finely chopped (optional)

Method:

1. Place a small skillet over medium heat. Add oil. When the oil is heated, add garlic and sauté until golden brown.

2. Stir in the mushrooms and cook until dry.

3. Meanwhile, add eggs and yogurt into a bowl and whisk well.

4. Remove half the mushrooms from the skillet and set aside.

5. Pour half the egg mixture into the pan and do not stir. Cook until the underside is cooked, as per your liking. Flip sides and cook the other side for a minute.

6.   Sprinkle half the chervil on top. Fold and serve.

7. Repeat with the mushrooms that were kept aside and with the remaining egg mixture.

Warm Chicken Salad

Serves: 4

Ingredients:

- [ ] 4 small chicken breasts, boneless, skinless, halved
- [ ] 2 large orange or red bell peppers, deseeded and cut into 1-inch squares
- [ ] 3 1/2 ounces watercress, tough stalks discarded
- [ ] 2/3 cucumber, sliced
- [ ] Juice of a small lemon
- [ ] Calorie-controlled cooking oil spray
- [ ] 2 little gem lettuce leaves, separated
- [ ] 4 ripe medium tomatoes, chopped
- [ ] 2 teaspoons thick balsamic vinegar

☐ Sea salt to taste

☐ Freshly ground black pepper to taste

Method:

1. Sprinkle salt and pepper all over the chicken.

2. Place a large nonstick pan over high heat. Spray some cooking spray over it.

3. Place chicken pieces in the pan and cook for 3 minutes. Flip sides and cook for 3 minutes or until tender inside. Remove with a slotted spoon and place on your cutting board. When cool enough to handle, slice the chicken.

4. Spray the pan again with a little oil. Add peppers and sauté until slight blisters appear on the skin.

5. Divide and place lettuce leaves on 4 serving plates. Sprinkle watercress, cucumber, tomatoes, and roasted peppers equally over them.

6. Divide and place chicken slices over the salad.

7. Trickle 1/2 teaspoon vinegar on each plate. Drizzle lemon juice on top. Sprinkle pepper on top and serve.

Lentil, Feta and Cherry Tomato Salad

Serves: 2

Ingredients:

- ☐ 3 1/2 ounces canned brown or green lentils, drained, rinsed

- ☐ 8 cherry tomatoes, halved

- ☐ 2 teaspoons lemon juice

- ☐ 2 teaspoons balsamic vinegar

- ☐ 3 1/2 ounces low-fat feta cheese, crumbled

- ☐ 3 1/2 ounces cucumber, chopped

- ☐ 4 spring onions, finely chopped

- ☐ A handful of fresh mint leaves, chopped (optional)

Method:

1. Add all the ingredients into a bowl and toss well.

2. Serve.

Spicy Beetroot and Coconut Soup with Herby Yogurt

Serves: 3

Ingredients:

For spice paste:

- [ ] 1 stalk lemongrass

- [ ] 1-2 red chilis, deseeded if desired

- [ ] 2 kaffir lime leaves

- [ ] 1 clove garlic, peeled

- [ ] 1 inch fresh ginger, peeled

- [ ] Juice of half a lime

For soup:

- [ ] 1/2 tablespoon vegetable oil

- [ ] Sea salt to taste

- [ ] 8.8 ounces cooked beets, peeled, chopped

- [ ] 7 ounces canned light coconut milk

- [ ] 1 banana shallot or 2 round shallots, finely chopped

- [ ] 1/2 teaspoon cumin seeds

- [ ] 1 cup vegetable stock

- [ ] Freshly ground pepper to taste

<u>For herby yogurt:</u>

- ☐ 1/2 tablespoon fresh cilantro, chopped

- ☐ 1/2 tablespoon fresh mint, chopped

- ☐ Flatbread to serve

- ☐ 1 tablespoon plain yogurt

- ☐ 1-inch sliced cucumber, chopped

Method:

1. To make spice paste: Add all the ingredients of the spice paste into a blender and blend until smooth. Sprinkle a little water if necessary.

2. To make soup: Place a soup pot over medium heat. Add oil. When the oil is heated, add cumin seeds. When the seeds crackle, add shallots and salt and sauté until tender.

3. Stir in the ground spice paste. Sauté for 3-4 minutes until aromatic.

4. Stir in the beets and sauté for a couple of minutes.

5. Add stock and stir. When it begins to boil, lower the heat and simmer for 5-7 minutes. Turn off the heat. Cool for a while.

6. Meanwhile, make the herby yogurt as follows: Add all the ingredients for herby yogurt into a bowl and stir. Set aside for a while for the flavors to set in.

7. Just before serving, transfer the soup into a blender. Add the coconut milk and blend again.

8. Pour soup back into the pot. Add salt and pepper and heat the soup.

9. Ladle into soup bowls. Drizzle some herby yogurt and serve along with flatbread.

Miso Broth

Serves: 2

Ingredients:

- ☐ 3-4 tablespoons miso paste

- ☐ 2 tablespoons dark soy sauce + extra to garnish

- ☐ 1 inch fresh ginger, peeled, grated

- ☐ 1 carrot, peeled, cut into matchsticks

- ☐ 3 1/2 ounces shiitake mushrooms, sliced

- ☐ 2 teaspoons mirin (rice wine)

- ☐ 2 teaspoons nam pla (Thai fish sauce)

- ☐ 3 1/2 ounces spring greens or savoy cabbage, thinly sliced

- ☐ 3 1/2 ounces beansprouts

- ☐ 4 cups water

Method:

1. Pour water into a soup pot. Place the pot over medium heat.

2. Add the rest of the ingredients and stir until the miso paste and nam pla are well combined. When it begins to boil, let it simmer for 5-6 minutes.

3. Ladle into soup bowls. Drizzle soy sauce on top and serve.

Chermoula Tofu and Roasted Red Vegetables

Serves: 2

Ingredients:

- ☐ A handful fresh cilantro, finely chopped

- ☐ 1/2 teaspoon cumin seeds, lightly crushed

- ☐ 1/4 teaspoon dried crushed chilis

- ☐ 4.5 ounces tofu, patted dried, cut into thin slices horizontally

- ☐ 1-2 cloves garlic, chopped

- ☐ Zest of 1/2 lemon, finely grated

- ☐ 1/2 tablespoon olive oil

For roasted vegetables:

- ☐ 1 red onion, quartered

- ☐ 1 yellow bell pepper, deseeded

- ☐ 1 red pepper, deseeded, sliced

- ☐ 1 zucchini, thickly sliced

- ☐ A pinch salt

- ☐ 1/2 small eggplant, thickly sliced

- ☐ Low-calorie cooking spray

Method:

1. To make chermoula: Add cilantro, cumin, dried chili, garlic, zest, and olive oil into a bowl and mix well.

2. Spread a generous amount of this mixture over the tofu slices.

3. To make roasted vegetables: Spread the vegetables in a baking pan. Spray with cooking spray.

4. Bake in a preheated oven at 390°F for 45 minutes or until slightly charred. Flip the vegetables a couple of times while baking.

5. Place the tofu slices over the vegetables with the chermoula side facing up. Bake for another 10-15 minutes.

6. Divide the tofu slices, along with the roasted vegetables, onto 2 plates and serve.

Stir-Fried Pork with Ginger and Soy Sauce

Serves: 4

Ingredients:

- [ ] 18 ounces pork tenderloin, trimmed of fat, chopped into chunks

- [ ] 4 tablespoons dark soy sauce

- [ ] 11 ounces button mushrooms, sliced

- [ ] 5 ounces snow pea, trimmed

- [ ] 2 cloves garlic, thinly sliced

- [ ] Freshly ground pepper to taste

- [ ] 2 teaspoons corn flour

- [ ] Low-calorie cooking spray

- [ ] 4 red peppers, deseeded, sliced

- [ ] 1 ounce fresh ginger, peeled, cut into matchsticks

- [ ] 8 spring onions, cut into 2-inch pieces

Method:

1. Sprinkle pepper all over the pork. Add corn flour into a bowl. Add 4 tablespoons cold water and mix well. Add soy sauce and mix well.

2. Place a large wok over high heat. Spray with cooking spray. Add pork and sauté for a couple of minutes until light brown but it should not be cooked thoroughly.

3. Remove with a slotted spoon and place on a plate.

4. Spray some more oil in the wok. Lower the heat to medium heat.

5. Add pepper and mushrooms and pepper and sauté for 2-3 minutes. Stir in the snow pea and sauté for a minute.

6. Stir in the garlic, ginger, and spring onions and sauté for a few seconds until fragrant.

7. Add pork back into the wok. Mix well. Stir in the corn flour mixture. Stir constantly until thick.

8. Serve.

Lamb and Flageolet Bean Stew

Serves: 8

Ingredients:

- ☐ 2 teaspoons olive oil

- ☐ 32 pickling onions

- ☐ 40 ounces lamb stock

- ☐ 1 large bouquet garni

- ☐ 22 ounces green beans

- ☐ Freshly ground pepper to taste

- ☐ 24 ounces lean lamb, cut into cubes

- ☐ 2 cloves garlic, crushed

- ☐ 1 can (14.5 ounces) chopped tomatoes

- ☐ 4 cans (14.5 ounces each) flageolet beans, drained, rinsed

- ☐ 18 ounces cherry tomatoes

Method:

1. Place a heatproof casserole dish over medium heat. Add oil. When the oil is heated, add lamb and sauté until brown.

2. Remove with a slotted spoon and set aside in a bowl.

3. Add garlic and onion into the casserole dish and sauté until onions turn light brown.

4. Add the lamb, tomatoes, beans, stock, and bouquet garni. When it begins to boil, lower the heat and cover with a lid. Simmer until lamb is tender.

5. Meanwhile, place a saucepan with water over medium heat. When the water begins to boil, add green beans and blanch for about a minute. Drain and immerse in ice-cold water for a couple of minutes. Drain and set aside.

6. Stir the cherry tomatoes into the simmering stew. Add pepper and simmer for 10-15 minutes.

7. Divide into bowls. Serve with green beans on the side.

Baked Apple with Crème Fraiche

Serves: 2

Ingredients:

- ☐ 2 large baking apples, cored

- ☐ 2 dessert spoon oats

- ☐ 2 teaspoons sultanas

- ☐ 2 teaspoons pumpkin seeds

- ☐ 4 tablespoons crème fraiche

- ☐ 2 teaspoons blanched almonds, to top

- ☐ 6 tablespoons apple juice

- ☐ 2 teaspoons vanilla extract

Method:

1. Add oats, sultanas, and pumpkin seeds into a bowl. Pour apple juice over them. Let soak for 20 minutes.

2. Add crème fraiche and vanilla into a bowl and stir.

3. Divide the soaked sultana mixture equally and fill in the core of the apple.

4. Sprinkle almonds on top.

5. Bake in a preheated oven at 300°F for 45-60 minutes.

6. Serve warm with crème fraiche.

Peppered Beef with Salad Leaves

Serves: 4

Ingredients:

- ☐ 4 thick-cut sirloin steaks (about 3 ounces each), trimmed of fat

- ☐ Coarse salt flakes to taste

- ☐ 1 teaspoon horseradish sauce

- ☐ 4 ounces mixed green salad leaves

- ☐ 1 red onion, thinly sliced

- ☐ Salt to taste

- ☐ Freshly ground pepper to taste

- ☐ 2 teaspoons colored peppercorns, coarsely crushed

- ☐ 4 1/2 ounces natural yogurt

- ☐ 1 clove garlic, crushed

- ☐ 2 1/2 ounces button mushrooms, sliced

☐   2 teaspoons olive oil

Method:

1. Sprinkle crushed peppercorns and salt flakes over the steaks and rub it into it.

2. Add yogurt, garlic, salt, freshly ground pepper, and horseradish sauce into a large bowl and mix well.

3. Toss in the salad leaves, mushrooms and ¾ the red onions.

4. Place a pan over high heat. Add oil. When the oil is heated, add steaks and sauté until brown.

5. Flip sides and cook the other side for 2 minutes, if you want it cooked medium rare, or 3-4 minutes for medium or 5 minutes for well-cooked. Cut into thin slices.

6. Remove steak and place on a plate.

7. Divide the salad into 4 plates. Place steak on top. Sprinkle remaining onions on top and serve.

Conclusion

I want to thank you once again for purchasing this book. I hope it proved to be an informative and an enjoyable read.

All the information that you need to create and follow an intermittent fasting plan that best suits your requirements is provided in this book. Try the different variations of this diet until you find one that works well for you. Intermittent fasting is not merely a diet; it is more of a lifestyle. If you want to lose weight in a sustainable manner and lose fat along with it, then this is the best diet for you. You can see a positive change in your body within four weeks when you follow this diet. Intermittent fasting concentrates on when you eat and not what you eat.

By now, you probably have realized the various benefits of this diet and how easy it is to follow as well. You need to make a couple of simple lifestyle changes and then you can reap all the benefits this diet offers. The recipes provided in this book are simple to understand and easy to follow. Follow these easy recipes to cook delicious food that is healthy and nutritious. Well, now all that you need to do is get started.

Thank you, and all the best!

Sources

https://caloriebee.com/diets/How-to-Lose-Weight-and-Eat-Healthy-on-a-Budget

http://paleoforwomen.com/shattering-the-myth-of-fasting-for-women-a-review-of-female-specific-responses-to-fasting-in-the-literature/#

https://blog.kettleandfire.com/intermittent-fasting-for-women/

https://www.precisionnutrition.com/intermittent-fasting-women

https://www.healthline.com/nutrition/10-health-benefits-of-intermittent-fasting#section7

https://www.popsugar.com/fitness/Types-Intermittent-Fasting-44871607

https://www.marksdailyapple.com/women-and-intermittent-fasting/